THIS BOOK BELONGS TO :

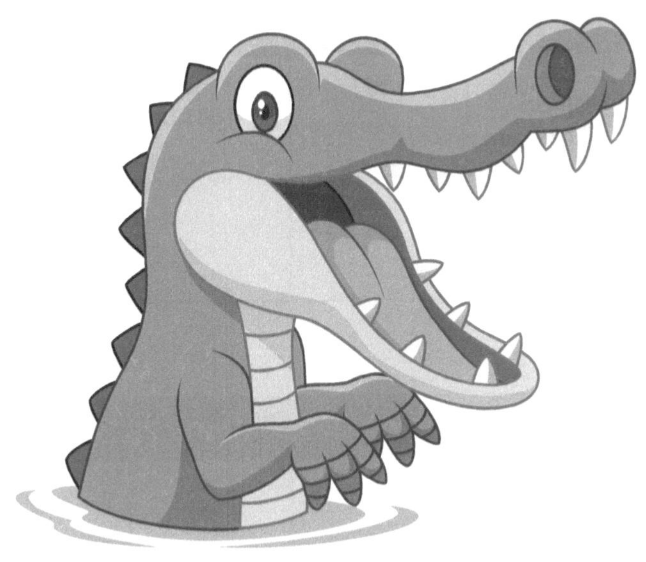

Date	Test	Breakfast	Lunch	Dinner	Bedtime
	Blood Pressure	/	/	/	/
	Blood Sugar				

Date	Test	Breakfast	Lunch	Dinner	Bedtime
	Blood Pressure	/	/	/	/
	Blood Sugar				

Date	Test	Breakfast	Lunch	Dinner	Bedtime
	Blood Pressure	/	/	/	/
	Blood Sugar				

Date	Test	Breakfast	Lunch	Dinner	Bedtime
	Blood Pressure	/	/	/	/
	Blood Sugar				

Date	Test	Breakfast	Lunch	Dinner	Bedtime
	Blood Pressure	/	/	/	/
	Blood Sugar				

Date	Test	Breakfast	Lunch	Dinner	Bedtime
	Blood Pressure	/	/	/	/
	Blood Sugar				

Date	Test	Breakfast	Lunch	Dinner	Bedtime
	Blood Pressure	/	/	/	/
	Blood Sugar				

Date	Test	Breakfast	Lunch	Dinner	Bedtime
	Blood Pressure	/	/	/	/
	Blood Sugar				

Date	Test	Breakfast	Lunch	Dinner	Bedtime
	Blood Pressure	/	/	/	/
	Blood Sugar				

Date	Test	Breakfast	Lunch	Dinner	Bedtime
	Blood Pressure	/	/	/	/
	Blood Sugar				

Date	Test	Breakfast	Lunch	Dinner	Bedtime
	Blood Pressure	/	/	/	/
	Blood Sugar				

Date	Test	Breakfast	Lunch	Dinner	Bedtime
	Blood Pressure	/	/	/	/
	Blood Sugar				

Date	Test	Breakfast	Lunch	Dinner	Bedtime
	Blood Pressure	/	/	/	/
	Blood Sugar				

Date	Test	Breakfast	Lunch	Dinner	Bedtime
	Blood Pressure	/	/	/	/
	Blood Sugar				

Date	Test	Breakfast	Lunch	Dinner	Bedtime
	Blood Pressure	/	/	/	/
	Blood Sugar				

Date	Test	Breakfast	Lunch	Dinner	Bedtime
	Blood Pressure	/	/	/	/
	Blood Sugar				

Date	Test	Breakfast	Lunch	Dinner	Bedtime
	Blood Pressure	/	/	/	/
	Blood Sugar				

Date	Test	Breakfast	Lunch	Dinner	Bedtime
	Blood Pressure	/	/	/	/
	Blood Sugar				

Date	Test	Breakfast	Lunch	Dinner	Bedtime
	Blood Pressure	/	/	/	/
	Blood Sugar				

Date	Test	Breakfast	Lunch	Dinner	Bedtime
	Blood Pressure	/	/	/	/
	Blood Sugar				

Date	Test	Breakfast	Lunch	Dinner	Bedtime
	Blood Pressure	/	/	/	/
	Blood Sugar				

Date	Test	Breakfast	Lunch	Dinner	Bedtime
	Blood Pressure	/	/	/	/
	Blood Sugar				

Date	Test	Breakfast	Lunch	Dinner	Bedtime
	Blood Pressure	/	/	/	/
	Blood Sugar				

Date	Test	Breakfast	Lunch	Dinner	Bedtime
	Blood Pressure	/	/	/	/
	Blood Sugar				

Date	Test	Breakfast	Lunch	Dinner	Bedtime
	Blood Pressure	/	/	/	/
	Blood Sugar				

Date	Test	Breakfast	Lunch	Dinner	Bedtime
	Blood Pressure	/	/	/	/
	Blood Sugar				

Date	Test	Breakfast	Lunch	Dinner	Bedtime
	Blood Pressure	/	/	/	/
	Blood Sugar				

Date	Test	Breakfast	Lunch	Dinner	Bedtime
	Blood Pressure	/	/	/	/
	Blood Sugar				

Date	Test	Breakfast	Lunch	Dinner	Bedtime
	Blood Pressure	/	/	/	/
	Blood Sugar				

Date	Test	Breakfast	Lunch	Dinner	Bedtime
	Blood Pressure	/	/	/	/
	Blood Sugar				

Date	Test	Breakfast	Lunch	Dinner	Bedtime
	Blood Pressure	/	/	/	/
	Blood Sugar				

Date	Test	Breakfast	Lunch	Dinner	Bedtime
	Blood Pressure	/	/	/	/
	Blood Sugar				

Date	Test	Breakfast	Lunch	Dinner	Bedtime
	Blood Pressure	/	/	/	/
	Blood Sugar				

Date	Test	Breakfast	Lunch	Dinner	Bedtime
	Blood Pressure	/	/	/	/
	Blood Sugar				

Date	Test	Breakfast	Lunch	Dinner	Bedtime
	Blood Pressure	/	/	/	/
	Blood Sugar				

Date	Test	Breakfast	Lunch	Dinner	Bedtime
	Blood Pressure	/	/	/	/
	Blood Sugar				

Date	Test	Breakfast	Lunch	Dinner	Bedtime
	Blood Pressure	/	/	/	/
	Blood Sugar				

Date	Test	Breakfast	Lunch	Dinner	Bedtime
	Blood Pressure	/	/	/	/
	Blood Sugar				

Date	Test	Breakfast	Lunch	Dinner	Bedtime
	Blood Pressure	/	/	/	/
	Blood Sugar				

Date	Test	Breakfast	Lunch	Dinner	Bedtime
	Blood Pressure	/	/	/	/
	Blood Sugar				

Date	Test	Breakfast	Lunch	Dinner	Bedtime
	Blood Pressure				
	Blood Sugar				

Date	Test	Breakfast	Lunch	Dinner	Bedtime
	Blood Pressure				
	Blood Sugar				

Date	Test	Breakfast	Lunch	Dinner	Bedtime
	Blood Pressure				
	Blood Sugar				

Date	Test	Breakfast	Lunch	Dinner	Bedtime
	Blood Pressure				
	Blood Sugar				

Date	Test	Breakfast	Lunch	Dinner	Bedtime
	Blood Pressure	/	/	/	/
	Blood Sugar				

Date	Test	Breakfast	Lunch	Dinner	Bedtime
	Blood Pressure	/	/	/	/
	Blood Sugar				

Date	Test	Breakfast	Lunch	Dinner	Bedtime
	Blood Pressure	/	/	/	/
	Blood Sugar				

Date	Test	Breakfast	Lunch	Dinner	Bedtime
	Blood Pressure	/	/	/	/
	Blood Sugar				

Date	Test	Breakfast	Lunch	Dinner	Bedtime
	Blood Pressure	/	/	/	/
	Blood Sugar				

Date	Test	Breakfast	Lunch	Dinner	Bedtime
	Blood Pressure	/	/	/	/
	Blood Sugar				

Date	Test	Breakfast	Lunch	Dinner	Bedtime
	Blood Pressure	/	/	/	/
	Blood Sugar				

Date	Test	Breakfast	Lunch	Dinner	Bedtime
	Blood Pressure	/	/	/	/
	Blood Sugar				

Date	Test	Breakfast	Lunch	Dinner	Bedtime
	Blood Pressure	/	/	/	/
	Blood Sugar				

Date	Test	Breakfast	Lunch	Dinner	Bedtime
	Blood Pressure	/	/	/	/
	Blood Sugar				

Date	Test	Breakfast	Lunch	Dinner	Bedtime
	Blood Pressure	/	/	/	/
	Blood Sugar				

Date	Test	Breakfast	Lunch	Dinner	Bedtime
	Blood Pressure	/	/	/	/
	Blood Sugar				

Date	Test	Breakfast	Lunch	Dinner	Bedtime
	Blood Pressure	/	/	/	/
	Blood Sugar				

Date	Test	Breakfast	Lunch	Dinner	Bedtime
	Blood Pressure	/	/	/	/
	Blood Sugar				

Date	Test	Breakfast	Lunch	Dinner	Bedtime
	Blood Pressure	/	/	/	/
	Blood Sugar				

Date	Test	Breakfast	Lunch	Dinner	Bedtime
	Blood Pressure	/	/	/	/
	Blood Sugar				

Date	Test	Breakfast	Lunch	Dinner	Bedtime
	Blood Pressure	/	/	/	/
	Blood Sugar				

Date	Test	Breakfast	Lunch	Dinner	Bedtime
	Blood Pressure	/	/	/	/
	Blood Sugar				

Date	Test	Breakfast	Lunch	Dinner	Bedtime
	Blood Pressure	/	/	/	/
	Blood Sugar				

Date	Test	Breakfast	Lunch	Dinner	Bedtime
	Blood Pressure	/	/	/	/
	Blood Sugar				

Date	Test	Breakfast	Lunch	Dinner	Bedtime
	Blood Pressure	/	/	/	/
	Blood Sugar				

Date	Test	Breakfast	Lunch	Dinner	Bedtime
	Blood Pressure	/	/	/	/
	Blood Sugar				

Date	Test	Breakfast	Lunch	Dinner	Bedtime
	Blood Pressure	/	/	/	/
	Blood Sugar				

Date	Test	Breakfast	Lunch	Dinner	Bedtime
	Blood Pressure	/	/	/	/
	Blood Sugar				

Date	Test	Breakfast	Lunch	Dinner	Bedtime
	Blood Pressure	/	/	/	/
	Blood Sugar				

Date	Test	Breakfast	Lunch	Dinner	Bedtime
	Blood Pressure	/	/	/	/
	Blood Sugar				

Date	Test	Breakfast	Lunch	Dinner	Bedtime
	Blood Pressure	/	/	/	/
	Blood Sugar				

Date	Test	Breakfast	Lunch	Dinner	Bedtime
	Blood Pressure	/	/	/	/
	Blood Sugar				

Date	Test	Breakfast	Lunch	Dinner	Bedtime
	Blood Pressure	/	/	/	/
	Blood Sugar				

Date	Test	Breakfast	Lunch	Dinner	Bedtime
	Blood Pressure	/	/	/	/
	Blood Sugar				

Date	Test	Breakfast	Lunch	Dinner	Bedtime
	Blood Pressure	/	/	/	/
	Blood Sugar				

Date	Test	Breakfast	Lunch	Dinner	Bedtime
	Blood Pressure	/	/	/	/
	Blood Sugar				

Date	Test	Breakfast	Lunch	Dinner	Bedtime
	Blood Pressure	/	/	/	/
	Blood Sugar				

Date	Test	Breakfast	Lunch	Dinner	Bedtime
	Blood Pressure	/	/	/	/
	Blood Sugar				

Date	Test	Breakfast	Lunch	Dinner	Bedtime
	Blood Pressure	/	/	/	/
	Blood Sugar				

Date	Test	Breakfast	Lunch	Dinner	Bedtime
	Blood Pressure	/	/	/	/
	Blood Sugar				

Date	Test	Breakfast	Lunch	Dinner	Bedtime
	Blood Pressure	/	/	/	/
	Blood Sugar				

Date	Test	Breakfast	Lunch	Dinner	Bedtime
	Blood Pressure	/	/	/	/
	Blood Sugar				

Date	Test	Breakfast	Lunch	Dinner	Bedtime
	Blood Pressure	/	/	/	/
	Blood Sugar				

Date	Test	Breakfast	Lunch	Dinner	Bedtime
	Blood Pressure	/	/	/	/
	Blood Sugar				

Date	Test	Breakfast	Lunch	Dinner	Bedtime
	Blood Pressure				
	Blood Sugar				

Date	Test	Breakfast	Lunch	Dinner	Bedtime
	Blood Pressure				
	Blood Sugar				

Date	Test	Breakfast	Lunch	Dinner	Bedtime
	Blood Pressure				
	Blood Sugar				

Date	Test	Breakfast	Lunch	Dinner	Bedtime
	Blood Pressure				
	Blood Sugar				

Date	Test	Breakfast	Lunch	Dinner	Bedtime
	Blood Pressure	/	/	/	/
	Blood Sugar				

Date	Test	Breakfast	Lunch	Dinner	Bedtime
	Blood Pressure	/	/	/	/
	Blood Sugar				

Date	Test	Breakfast	Lunch	Dinner	Bedtime
	Blood Pressure	/	/	/	/
	Blood Sugar				

Date	Test	Breakfast	Lunch	Dinner	Bedtime
	Blood Pressure	/	/	/	/
	Blood Sugar				

Date	Test	Breakfast	Lunch	Dinner	Bedtime
	Blood Pressure	/	/	/	/
	Blood Sugar				

Date	Test	Breakfast	Lunch	Dinner	Bedtime
	Blood Pressure	/	/	/	/
	Blood Sugar				

Date	Test	Breakfast	Lunch	Dinner	Bedtime
	Blood Pressure	/	/	/	/
	Blood Sugar				

Date	Test	Breakfast	Lunch	Dinner	Bedtime
	Blood Pressure	/	/	/	/
	Blood Sugar				

Date	Test	Breakfast	Lunch	Dinner	Bedtime
	Blood Pressure	/	/	/	/
	Blood Sugar				

Date	Test	Breakfast	Lunch	Dinner	Bedtime
	Blood Pressure	/	/	/	/
	Blood Sugar				

Date	Test	Breakfast	Lunch	Dinner	Bedtime
	Blood Pressure	/	/	/	/
	Blood Sugar				

Date	Test	Breakfast	Lunch	Dinner	Bedtime
	Blood Pressure	/	/	/	/
	Blood Sugar				

Date	Test	Breakfast	Lunch	Dinner	Bedtime
	Blood Pressure	/	/	/	/
	Blood Sugar				

Date	Test	Breakfast	Lunch	Dinner	Bedtime
	Blood Pressure	/	/	/	/
	Blood Sugar				

Date	Test	Breakfast	Lunch	Dinner	Bedtime
	Blood Pressure	/	/	/	/
	Blood Sugar				

Date	Test	Breakfast	Lunch	Dinner	Bedtime
	Blood Pressure	/	/	/	/
	Blood Sugar				

Date	Test	Breakfast	Lunch	Dinner	Bedtime
	Blood Pressure	/	/	/	/
	Blood Sugar				

Date	Test	Breakfast	Lunch	Dinner	Bedtime
	Blood Pressure	/	/	/	/
	Blood Sugar				

Date	Test	Breakfast	Lunch	Dinner	Bedtime
	Blood Pressure	/	/	/	/
	Blood Sugar				

Date	Test	Breakfast	Lunch	Dinner	Bedtime
	Blood Pressure	/	/	/	/
	Blood Sugar				

Date	Test	Breakfast	Lunch	Dinner	Bedtime
	Blood Pressure	/	/	/	/
	Blood Sugar				

Date	Test	Breakfast	Lunch	Dinner	Bedtime
	Blood Pressure	/	/	/	/
	Blood Sugar				

Date	Test	Breakfast	Lunch	Dinner	Bedtime
	Blood Pressure	/	/	/	/
	Blood Sugar				

Date	Test	Breakfast	Lunch	Dinner	Bedtime
	Blood Pressure	/	/	/	/
	Blood Sugar				

Date	Test	Breakfast	Lunch	Dinner	Bedtime
	Blood Pressure	/	/	/	/
	Blood Sugar				

Date	Test	Breakfast	Lunch	Dinner	Bedtime
	Blood Pressure	/	/	/	/
	Blood Sugar				

Date	Test	Breakfast	Lunch	Dinner	Bedtime
	Blood Pressure	/	/	/	/
	Blood Sugar				

Date	Test	Breakfast	Lunch	Dinner	Bedtime
	Blood Pressure	/	/	/	/
	Blood Sugar				

Date	Test	Breakfast	Lunch	Dinner	Bedtime
	Blood Pressure	/	/	/	/
	Blood Sugar				

Date	Test	Breakfast	Lunch	Dinner	Bedtime
	Blood Pressure	/	/	/	/
	Blood Sugar				

Date	Test	Breakfast	Lunch	Dinner	Bedtime
	Blood Pressure	/	/	/	/
	Blood Sugar				

Date	Test	Breakfast	Lunch	Dinner	Bedtime
	Blood Pressure	/	/	/	/
	Blood Sugar				

Date	Test	Breakfast	Lunch	Dinner	Bedtime
	Blood Pressure	/	/	/	/
	Blood Sugar				

Date	Test	Breakfast	Lunch	Dinner	Bedtime
	Blood Pressure	/	/	/	/
	Blood Sugar				

Date	Test	Breakfast	Lunch	Dinner	Bedtime
	Blood Pressure	/	/	/	/
	Blood Sugar				

Date	Test	Breakfast	Lunch	Dinner	Bedtime
	Blood Pressure	/	/	/	/
	Blood Sugar				

Date	Test	Breakfast	Lunch	Dinner	Bedtime
	Blood Pressure	/	/	/	/
	Blood Sugar				

Date	Test	Breakfast	Lunch	Dinner	Bedtime
	Blood Pressure	/	/	/	/
	Blood Sugar				

Date	Test	Breakfast	Lunch	Dinner	Bedtime
	Blood Pressure	/	/	/	/
	Blood Sugar				

Date	Test	Breakfast	Lunch	Dinner	Bedtime
	Blood Pressure	/	/	/	/
	Blood Sugar				

Date	Test	Breakfast	Lunch	Dinner	Bedtime
	Blood Pressure	/	/	/	/
	Blood Sugar				

Date	Test	Breakfast	Lunch	Dinner	Bedtime
	Blood Pressure	/	/	/	/
	Blood Sugar				

Date	Test	Breakfast	Lunch	Dinner	Bedtime
	Blood Pressure	/	/	/	/
	Blood Sugar				

Date	Test	Breakfast	Lunch	Dinner	Bedtime
	Blood Pressure	/	/	/	/
	Blood Sugar				

Date	Test	Breakfast	Lunch	Dinner	Bedtime
	Blood Pressure	/	/	/	/
	Blood Sugar				

Date	Test	Breakfast	Lunch	Dinner	Bedtime
	Blood Pressure	/	/	/	/
	Blood Sugar				

Date	Test	Breakfast	Lunch	Dinner	Bedtime
	Blood Pressure	/	/	/	/
	Blood Sugar				

Date	Test	Breakfast	Lunch	Dinner	Bedtime
	Blood Pressure	/	/	/	/
	Blood Sugar				

Date	Test	Breakfast	Lunch	Dinner	Bedtime
	Blood Pressure	/	/	/	/
	Blood Sugar				

Date	Test	Breakfast	Lunch	Dinner	Bedtime
	Blood Pressure	/	/	/	/
	Blood Sugar				

Date	Test	Breakfast	Lunch	Dinner	Bedtime
	Blood Pressure	/	/	/	/
	Blood Sugar				

Date	Test	Breakfast	Lunch	Dinner	Bedtime
	Blood Pressure	/	/	/	/
	Blood Sugar				

Date	Test	Breakfast	Lunch	Dinner	Bedtime
	Blood Pressure	/	/	/	/
	Blood Sugar				

Date	Test	Breakfast	Lunch	Dinner	Bedtime
	Blood Pressure	/	/	/	/
	Blood Sugar				

Date	Test	Breakfast	Lunch	Dinner	Bedtime
	Blood Pressure	/	/	/	/
	Blood Sugar				

Date	Test	Breakfast	Lunch	Dinner	Bedtime
	Blood Pressure	/	/	/	/
	Blood Sugar				

Date	Test	Breakfast	Lunch	Dinner	Bedtime
	Blood Pressure	/	/	/	/
	Blood Sugar				

Date	Test	Breakfast	Lunch	Dinner	Bedtime
	Blood Pressure	/	/	/	/
	Blood Sugar				

Date	Test	Breakfast	Lunch	Dinner	Bedtime
	Blood Pressure	/	/	/	/
	Blood Sugar				

Date	Test	Breakfast	Lunch	Dinner	Bedtime
	Blood Pressure	/	/	/	/
	Blood Sugar				

Date	Test	Breakfast	Lunch	Dinner	Bedtime
	Blood Pressure	/	/	/	/
	Blood Sugar				

Date	Test	Breakfast	Lunch	Dinner	Bedtime
	Blood Pressure	/	/	/	/
	Blood Sugar				

Date	Test	Breakfast	Lunch	Dinner	Bedtime
	Blood Pressure	/	/	/	/
	Blood Sugar				

Date	Test	Breakfast	Lunch	Dinner	Bedtime
	Blood Pressure	/	/	/	/
	Blood Sugar				

Date	Test	Breakfast	Lunch	Dinner	Bedtime
	Blood Pressure	/	/	/	/
	Blood Sugar				

Date	Test	Breakfast	Lunch	Dinner	Bedtime
	Blood Pressure	/	/	/	/
	Blood Sugar				

Date	Test	Breakfast	Lunch	Dinner	Bedtime
	Blood Pressure	/	/	/	/
	Blood Sugar				

Date	Test	Breakfast	Lunch	Dinner	Bedtime
	Blood Pressure	/	/	/	/
	Blood Sugar				

Date	Test	Breakfast	Lunch	Dinner	Bedtime
	Blood Pressure	/	/	/	/
	Blood Sugar				

Date	Test	Breakfast	Lunch	Dinner	Bedtime
	Blood Pressure	/	/	/	/
	Blood Sugar				

Date	Test	Breakfast	Lunch	Dinner	Bedtime
	Blood Pressure	/	/	/	/
	Blood Sugar				

Date	Test	Breakfast	Lunch	Dinner	Bedtime
	Blood Pressure	/	/	/	/
	Blood Sugar				

Date	Test	Breakfast	Lunch	Dinner	Bedtime
	Blood Pressure	/	/	/	/
	Blood Sugar				

Date	Test	Breakfast	Lunch	Dinner	Bedtime
	Blood Pressure	/	/	/	/
	Blood Sugar				

Date	Test	Breakfast	Lunch	Dinner	Bedtime
	Blood Pressure	/	/	/	/
	Blood Sugar				

Date	Test	Breakfast	Lunch	Dinner	Bedtime
	Blood Pressure	/	/	/	/
	Blood Sugar				

Date	Test	Breakfast	Lunch	Dinner	Bedtime
	Blood Pressure	/	/	/	/
	Blood Sugar				

Date	Test	Breakfast	Lunch	Dinner	Bedtime
	Blood Pressure	/	/	/	/
	Blood Sugar				

Date	Test	Breakfast	Lunch	Dinner	Bedtime
	Blood Pressure	/	/	/	/
	Blood Sugar				

Date	Test	Breakfast	Lunch	Dinner	Bedtime
	Blood Pressure	/	/	/	/
	Blood Sugar				

Date	Test	Breakfast	Lunch	Dinner	Bedtime
	Blood Pressure	/	/	/	/
	Blood Sugar				

Date	Test	Breakfast	Lunch	Dinner	Bedtime
	Blood Pressure	/	/	/	/
	Blood Sugar				

Date	Test	Breakfast	Lunch	Dinner	Bedtime
	Blood Pressure	/	/	/	/
	Blood Sugar				

Date	Test	Breakfast	Lunch	Dinner	Bedtime
	Blood Pressure	/	/	/	/
	Blood Sugar				

Date	Test	Breakfast	Lunch	Dinner	Bedtime
	Blood Pressure	/	/	/	/
	Blood Sugar				

Date	Test	Breakfast	Lunch	Dinner	Bedtime
	Blood Pressure	/	/	/	/
	Blood Sugar				

Date	Test	Breakfast	Lunch	Dinner	Bedtime
	Blood Pressure	/	/	/	/
	Blood Sugar				

Date	Test	Breakfast	Lunch	Dinner	Bedtime
	Blood Pressure	/	/	/	/
	Blood Sugar				

Date	Test	Breakfast	Lunch	Dinner	Bedtime
	Blood Pressure	/	/	/	/
	Blood Sugar				

Date	Test	Breakfast	Lunch	Dinner	Bedtime
	Blood Pressure	/	/	/	/
	Blood Sugar				

Date	Test	Breakfast	Lunch	Dinner	Bedtime
	Blood Pressure	/	/	/	/
	Blood Sugar				

Date	Test	Breakfast	Lunch	Dinner	Bedtime
	Blood Pressure	/	/	/	/
	Blood Sugar				

Date	Test	Breakfast	Lunch	Dinner	Bedtime
	Blood Pressure	/	/	/	/
	Blood Sugar				

Date	Test	Breakfast	Lunch	Dinner	Bedtime
	Blood Pressure	/	/	/	/
	Blood Sugar				

Date	Test	Breakfast	Lunch	Dinner	Bedtime
	Blood Pressure	/	/	/	/
	Blood Sugar				

Date	Test	Breakfast	Lunch	Dinner	Bedtime
	Blood Pressure	/	/	/	/
	Blood Sugar				

Date	Test	Breakfast	Lunch	Dinner	Bedtime
	Blood Pressure	/	/	/	/
	Blood Sugar				

Date	Test	Breakfast	Lunch	Dinner	Bedtime
	Blood Pressure	/	/	/	/
	Blood Sugar				

Date	Test	Breakfast	Lunch	Dinner	Bedtime
	Blood Pressure	/	/	/	/
	Blood Sugar				

Date	Test	Breakfast	Lunch	Dinner	Bedtime
	Blood Pressure	/	/	/	/
	Blood Sugar				

Date	Test	Breakfast	Lunch	Dinner	Bedtime
	Blood Pressure	/	/	/	/
	Blood Sugar				

Date	Test	Breakfast	Lunch	Dinner	Bedtime
	Blood Pressure	/	/	/	/
	Blood Sugar				

Date	Test	Breakfast	Lunch	Dinner	Bedtime
	Blood Pressure	/	/	/	/
	Blood Sugar				

Date	Test	Breakfast	Lunch	Dinner	Bedtime
	Blood Pressure	/	/	/	/
	Blood Sugar				

Date	Test	Breakfast	Lunch	Dinner	Bedtime
	Blood Pressure	/	/	/	/
	Blood Sugar				

Date	Test	Breakfast	Lunch	Dinner	Bedtime
	Blood Pressure	/	/	/	/
	Blood Sugar				

Date	Test	Breakfast	Lunch	Dinner	Bedtime
	Blood Pressure	/	/	/	/
	Blood Sugar				

Date	Test	Breakfast	Lunch	Dinner	Bedtime
	Blood Pressure	/	/	/	/
	Blood Sugar				

Date	Test	Breakfast	Lunch	Dinner	Bedtime
	Blood Pressure	/	/	/	/
	Blood Sugar				

Date	Test	Breakfast	Lunch	Dinner	Bedtime
	Blood Pressure	/	/	/	/
	Blood Sugar				

Date	Test	Breakfast	Lunch	Dinner	Bedtime
	Blood Pressure	/	/	/	/
	Blood Sugar				

Date	Test	Breakfast	Lunch	Dinner	Bedtime
	Blood Pressure	/	/	/	/
	Blood Sugar				

Date	Test	Breakfast	Lunch	Dinner	Bedtime
	Blood Pressure	/	/	/	/
	Blood Sugar				

Date	Test	Breakfast	Lunch	Dinner	Bedtime
	Blood Pressure	/	/	/	/
	Blood Sugar				

Date	Test	Breakfast	Lunch	Dinner	Bedtime
	Blood Pressure	/	/	/	/
	Blood Sugar				

Date	Test	Breakfast	Lunch	Dinner	Bedtime
	Blood Pressure	/	/	/	/
	Blood Sugar				

Date	Test	Breakfast	Lunch	Dinner	Bedtime
	Blood Pressure	/	/	/	/
	Blood Sugar				

Date	Test	Breakfast	Lunch	Dinner	Bedtime
	Blood Pressure	/	/	/	/
	Blood Sugar				

Date	Test	Breakfast	Lunch	Dinner	Bedtime
	Blood Pressure	/	/	/	/
	Blood Sugar				

Date	Test	Breakfast	Lunch	Dinner	Bedtime
	Blood Pressure	/	/	/	/
	Blood Sugar				

Date	Test	Breakfast	Lunch	Dinner	Bedtime
	Blood Pressure	/	/	/	/
	Blood Sugar				

Date	Test	Breakfast	Lunch	Dinner	Bedtime
	Blood Pressure	/	/	/	/
	Blood Sugar				

Date	Test	Breakfast	Lunch	Dinner	Bedtime
	Blood Pressure	/	/	/	/
	Blood Sugar				

Date	Test	Breakfast	Lunch	Dinner	Bedtime
	Blood Pressure	/	/	/	/
	Blood Sugar				

Date	Test	Breakfast	Lunch	Dinner	Bedtime
	Blood Pressure	/	/	/	/
	Blood Sugar				

Date	Test	Breakfast	Lunch	Dinner	Bedtime
	Blood Pressure	/	/	/	/
	Blood Sugar				

Date	Test	Breakfast	Lunch	Dinner	Bedtime
	Blood Pressure	/	/	/	/
	Blood Sugar				

Date	Test	Breakfast	Lunch	Dinner	Bedtime
	Blood Pressure	/	/	/	/
	Blood Sugar				

Date	Test	Breakfast	Lunch	Dinner	Bedtime
	Blood Pressure	/	/	/	/
	Blood Sugar				

Date	Test	Breakfast	Lunch	Dinner	Bedtime
	Blood Pressure	/	/	/	/
	Blood Sugar				

Date	Test	Breakfast	Lunch	Dinner	Bedtime
	Blood Pressure	/	/	/	/
	Blood Sugar				

Date	Test	Breakfast	Lunch	Dinner	Bedtime
	Blood Pressure	/	/	/	/
	Blood Sugar				

Date	Test	Breakfast	Lunch	Dinner	Bedtime
	Blood Pressure	/	/	/	/
	Blood Sugar				

Date	Test	Breakfast	Lunch	Dinner	Bedtime
	Blood Pressure	/	/	/	/
	Blood Sugar				

Date	Test	Breakfast	Lunch	Dinner	Bedtime
	Blood Pressure	/	/	/	/
	Blood Sugar				

Date	Test	Breakfast	Lunch	Dinner	Bedtime
	Blood Pressure	/	/	/	/
	Blood Sugar				

Date	Test	Breakfast	Lunch	Dinner	Bedtime
	Blood Pressure	/	/	/	/
	Blood Sugar				

Date	Test	Breakfast	Lunch	Dinner	Bedtime
	Blood Pressure	/	/	/	/
	Blood Sugar				

Date	Test	Breakfast	Lunch	Dinner	Bedtime
	Blood Pressure	/	/	/	/
	Blood Sugar				

Date	Test	Breakfast	Lunch	Dinner	Bedtime
	Blood Pressure	/	/	/	/
	Blood Sugar				

Date	Test	Breakfast	Lunch	Dinner	Bedtime
	Blood Pressure	/	/	/	/
	Blood Sugar				

Date	Test	Breakfast	Lunch	Dinner	Bedtime
	Blood Pressure	/	/	/	/
	Blood Sugar				

Date	Test	Breakfast	Lunch	Dinner	Bedtime
	Blood Pressure	/	/	/	/
	Blood Sugar				

Date	Test	Breakfast	Lunch	Dinner	Bedtime
	Blood Pressure	/	/	/	/
	Blood Sugar				

Date	Test	Breakfast	Lunch	Dinner	Bedtime
	Blood Pressure	/	/	/	/
	Blood Sugar				

Date	Test	Breakfast	Lunch	Dinner	Bedtime
	Blood Pressure	/	/	/	/
	Blood Sugar				

Date	Test	Breakfast	Lunch	Dinner	Bedtime
	Blood Pressure	/	/	/	/
	Blood Sugar				

Date	Test	Breakfast	Lunch	Dinner	Bedtime
	Blood Pressure	/	/	/	/
	Blood Sugar				

Date	Test	Breakfast	Lunch	Dinner	Bedtime
	Blood Pressure	/	/	/	/
	Blood Sugar				

Date	Test	Breakfast	Lunch	Dinner	Bedtime
	Blood Pressure	/	/	/	/
	Blood Sugar				

Date	Test	Breakfast	Lunch	Dinner	Bedtime
	Blood Pressure	/	/	/	/
	Blood Sugar				

Date	Test	Breakfast	Lunch	Dinner	Bedtime
	Blood Pressure	/	/	/	/
	Blood Sugar				

Date	Test	Breakfast	Lunch	Dinner	Bedtime
	Blood Pressure	/	/	/	/
	Blood Sugar				

Date	Test	Breakfast	Lunch	Dinner	Bedtime
	Blood Pressure	/	/	/	/
	Blood Sugar				

Date	Test	Breakfast	Lunch	Dinner	Bedtime
	Blood Pressure	/	/	/	/
	Blood Sugar				

Date	Test	Breakfast	Lunch	Dinner	Bedtime
	Blood Pressure	/	/	/	/
	Blood Sugar				

Date	Test	Breakfast	Lunch	Dinner	Bedtime
	Blood Pressure				
	Blood Sugar				

Date	Test	Breakfast	Lunch	Dinner	Bedtime
	Blood Pressure				
	Blood Sugar				

Date	Test	Breakfast	Lunch	Dinner	Bedtime
	Blood Pressure				
	Blood Sugar				

Date	Test	Breakfast	Lunch	Dinner	Bedtime
	Blood Pressure				
	Blood Sugar				

Date	Test	Breakfast	Lunch	Dinner	Bedtime
	Blood Pressure	/	/	/	/
	Blood Sugar				

Date	Test	Breakfast	Lunch	Dinner	Bedtime
	Blood Pressure	/	/	/	/
	Blood Sugar				

Date	Test	Breakfast	Lunch	Dinner	Bedtime
	Blood Pressure	/	/	/	/
	Blood Sugar				

Date	Test	Breakfast	Lunch	Dinner	Bedtime
	Blood Pressure	/	/	/	/
	Blood Sugar				

Date	Test	Breakfast	Lunch	Dinner	Bedtime
	Blood Pressure	/	/	/	/
	Blood Sugar				

Date	Test	Breakfast	Lunch	Dinner	Bedtime
	Blood Pressure	/	/	/	/
	Blood Sugar				

Date	Test	Breakfast	Lunch	Dinner	Bedtime
	Blood Pressure	/	/	/	/
	Blood Sugar				

Date	Test	Breakfast	Lunch	Dinner	Bedtime
	Blood Pressure	/	/	/	/
	Blood Sugar				

Date	Test	Breakfast	Lunch	Dinner	Bedtime
	Blood Pressure	/	/	/	/
	Blood Sugar				

Date	Test	Breakfast	Lunch	Dinner	Bedtime
	Blood Pressure	/	/	/	/
	Blood Sugar				

Date	Test	Breakfast	Lunch	Dinner	Bedtime
	Blood Pressure	/	/	/	/
	Blood Sugar				

Date	Test	Breakfast	Lunch	Dinner	Bedtime
	Blood Pressure	/	/	/	/
	Blood Sugar				

Date	Test	Breakfast	Lunch	Dinner	Bedtime
	Blood Pressure	/	/	/	/
	Blood Sugar				

Date	Test	Breakfast	Lunch	Dinner	Bedtime
	Blood Pressure	/	/	/	/
	Blood Sugar				

Date	Test	Breakfast	Lunch	Dinner	Bedtime
	Blood Pressure	/	/	/	/
	Blood Sugar				

Date	Test	Breakfast	Lunch	Dinner	Bedtime
	Blood Pressure	/	/	/	/
	Blood Sugar				

Date	Test	Breakfast	Lunch	Dinner	Bedtime
	Blood Pressure	/	/	/	/
	Blood Sugar				

Date	Test	Breakfast	Lunch	Dinner	Bedtime
	Blood Pressure	/	/	/	/
	Blood Sugar				

Date	Test	Breakfast	Lunch	Dinner	Bedtime
	Blood Pressure	/	/	/	/
	Blood Sugar				

Date	Test	Breakfast	Lunch	Dinner	Bedtime
	Blood Pressure	/	/	/	/
	Blood Sugar				

Date	Test	Breakfast	Lunch	Dinner	Bedtime
	Blood Pressure	/	/	/	/
	Blood Sugar				

Date	Test	Breakfast	Lunch	Dinner	Bedtime
	Blood Pressure	/	/	/	/
	Blood Sugar				

Date	Test	Breakfast	Lunch	Dinner	Bedtime
	Blood Pressure	/	/	/	/
	Blood Sugar				

Date	Test	Breakfast	Lunch	Dinner	Bedtime
	Blood Pressure	/	/	/	/
	Blood Sugar				

Date	Test	Breakfast	Lunch	Dinner	Bedtime
	Blood Pressure	/	/	/	/
	Blood Sugar				

Date	Test	Breakfast	Lunch	Dinner	Bedtime
	Blood Pressure	/	/	/	/
	Blood Sugar				

Date	Test	Breakfast	Lunch	Dinner	Bedtime
	Blood Pressure	/	/	/	/
	Blood Sugar				

Date	Test	Breakfast	Lunch	Dinner	Bedtime
	Blood Pressure	/	/	/	/
	Blood Sugar				

Date	Test	Breakfast	Lunch	Dinner	Bedtime
	Blood Pressure	/	/	/	/
	Blood Sugar				

Date	Test	Breakfast	Lunch	Dinner	Bedtime
	Blood Pressure	/	/	/	/
	Blood Sugar				

Date	Test	Breakfast	Lunch	Dinner	Bedtime
	Blood Pressure	/	/	/	/
	Blood Sugar				

Date	Test	Breakfast	Lunch	Dinner	Bedtime
	Blood Pressure	/	/	/	/
	Blood Sugar				

Date	Test	Breakfast	Lunch	Dinner	Bedtime
	Blood Pressure	/	/	/	/
	Blood Sugar				

Date	Test	Breakfast	Lunch	Dinner	Bedtime
	Blood Pressure	/	/	/	/
	Blood Sugar				

Date	Test	Breakfast	Lunch	Dinner	Bedtime
	Blood Pressure	/	/	/	/
	Blood Sugar				

Date	Test	Breakfast	Lunch	Dinner	Bedtime
	Blood Pressure	/	/	/	/
	Blood Sugar				

Date	Test	Breakfast	Lunch	Dinner	Bedtime
	Blood Pressure	/	/	/	/
	Blood Sugar				

Date	Test	Breakfast	Lunch	Dinner	Bedtime
	Blood Pressure	/	/	/	/
	Blood Sugar				

Date	Test	Breakfast	Lunch	Dinner	Bedtime
	Blood Pressure	/	/	/	/
	Blood Sugar				

Date	Test	Breakfast	Lunch	Dinner	Bedtime
	Blood Pressure	/	/	/	/
	Blood Sugar				

Date	Test	Breakfast	Lunch	Dinner	Bedtime
	Blood Pressure	/	/	/	/
	Blood Sugar				

Date	Test	Breakfast	Lunch	Dinner	Bedtime
	Blood Pressure	/	/	/	/
	Blood Sugar				

Date	Test	Breakfast	Lunch	Dinner	Bedtime
	Blood Pressure	/	/	/	/
	Blood Sugar				

Date	Test	Breakfast	Lunch	Dinner	Bedtime
	Blood Pressure	/	/	/	/
	Blood Sugar				

Date	Test	Breakfast	Lunch	Dinner	Bedtime
	Blood Pressure	/	/	/	/
	Blood Sugar				

Date	Test	Breakfast	Lunch	Dinner	Bedtime
	Blood Pressure	/	/	/	/
	Blood Sugar				

Date	Test	Breakfast	Lunch	Dinner	Bedtime
	Blood Pressure	/	/	/	/
	Blood Sugar				

Date	Test	Breakfast	Lunch	Dinner	Bedtime
	Blood Pressure	/	/	/	/
	Blood Sugar				

Date	Test	Breakfast	Lunch	Dinner	Bedtime
	Blood Pressure	/	/	/	/
	Blood Sugar				

Date	Test	Breakfast	Lunch	Dinner	Bedtime
	Blood Pressure	/	/	/	/
	Blood Sugar				

Date	Test	Breakfast	Lunch	Dinner	Bedtime
	Blood Pressure	/	/	/	/
	Blood Sugar				

Date	Test	Breakfast	Lunch	Dinner	Bedtime
	Blood Pressure	/	/	/	/
	Blood Sugar				

Date	Test	Breakfast	Lunch	Dinner	Bedtime
	Blood Pressure	/	/	/	/
	Blood Sugar				

Date	Test	Breakfast	Lunch	Dinner	Bedtime
	Blood Pressure	/	/	/	/
	Blood Sugar				

Date	Test	Breakfast	Lunch	Dinner	Bedtime
	Blood Pressure	/	/	/	/
	Blood Sugar				

Date	Test	Breakfast	Lunch	Dinner	Bedtime
	Blood Pressure	/	/	/	/
	Blood Sugar				

Date	Test	Breakfast	Lunch	Dinner	Bedtime
	Blood Pressure	/	/	/	/
	Blood Sugar				

Date	Test	Breakfast	Lunch	Dinner	Bedtime
	Blood Pressure	/	/	/	/
	Blood Sugar				

Date	Test	Breakfast	Lunch	Dinner	Bedtime
	Blood Pressure	/	/	/	/
	Blood Sugar				

Date	Test	Breakfast	Lunch	Dinner	Bedtime
	Blood Pressure	/	/	/	/
	Blood Sugar				

Date	Test	Breakfast	Lunch	Dinner	Bedtime
	Blood Pressure	/	/	/	/
	Blood Sugar				

Date	Test	Breakfast	Lunch	Dinner	Bedtime
	Blood Pressure	/	/	/	/
	Blood Sugar				

Date	Test	Breakfast	Lunch	Dinner	Bedtime
	Blood Pressure	/	/	/	/
	Blood Sugar				

Date	Test	Breakfast	Lunch	Dinner	Bedtime
	Blood Pressure	/	/	/	/
	Blood Sugar				

Date	Test	Breakfast	Lunch	Dinner	Bedtime
	Blood Pressure	/	/	/	/
	Blood Sugar				

Date	Test	Breakfast	Lunch	Dinner	Bedtime
	Blood Pressure	/	/	/	/
	Blood Sugar				

Date	Test	Breakfast	Lunch	Dinner	Bedtime
	Blood Pressure	/	/	/	/
	Blood Sugar				

Date	Test	Breakfast	Lunch	Dinner	Bedtime
	Blood Pressure	/	/	/	/
	Blood Sugar				

Date	Test	Breakfast	Lunch	Dinner	Bedtime
	Blood Pressure	/	/	/	/
	Blood Sugar				

Date	Test	Breakfast	Lunch	Dinner	Bedtime
	Blood Pressure	/	/	/	/
	Blood Sugar				

Date	Test	Breakfast	Lunch	Dinner	Bedtime
	Blood Pressure	/	/	/	/
	Blood Sugar				

Date	Test	Breakfast	Lunch	Dinner	Bedtime
	Blood Pressure	/	/	/	/
	Blood Sugar				

Date	Test	Breakfast	Lunch	Dinner	Bedtime
	Blood Pressure	/	/	/	/
	Blood Sugar				

Date	Test	Breakfast	Lunch	Dinner	Bedtime
	Blood Pressure	/	/	/	/
	Blood Sugar				

Date	Test	Breakfast	Lunch	Dinner	Bedtime
	Blood Pressure	/	/	/	/
	Blood Sugar				

Date	Test	Breakfast	Lunch	Dinner	Bedtime
	Blood Pressure	/	/	/	/
	Blood Sugar				

Date	Test	Breakfast	Lunch	Dinner	Bedtime
	Blood Pressure	/	/	/	/
	Blood Sugar				

Date	Test	Breakfast	Lunch	Dinner	Bedtime
	Blood Pressure	/	/	/	/
	Blood Sugar				

Date	Test	Breakfast	Lunch	Dinner	Bedtime
	Blood Pressure	/	/	/	/
	Blood Sugar				

Date	Test	Breakfast	Lunch	Dinner	Bedtime
	Blood Pressure	/	/	/	/
	Blood Sugar				

Date	Test	Breakfast	Lunch	Dinner	Bedtime
	Blood Pressure	/	/	/	/
	Blood Sugar				

Date	Test	Breakfast	Lunch	Dinner	Bedtime
	Blood Pressure	/	/	/	/
	Blood Sugar				

Date	Test	Breakfast	Lunch	Dinner	Bedtime
	Blood Pressure	/	/	/	/
	Blood Sugar				

Date	Test	Breakfast	Lunch	Dinner	Bedtime
	Blood Pressure	/	/	/	/
	Blood Sugar				

Date	Test	Breakfast	Lunch	Dinner	Bedtime
	Blood Pressure	/	/	/	/
	Blood Sugar				

Date	Test	Breakfast	Lunch	Dinner	Bedtime
	Blood Pressure	/	/	/	/
	Blood Sugar				

Date	Test	Breakfast	Lunch	Dinner	Bedtime
	Blood Pressure	/	/	/	/
	Blood Sugar				

Date	Test	Breakfast	Lunch	Dinner	Bedtime
	Blood Pressure	/	/	/	/
	Blood Sugar				

Date	Test	Breakfast	Lunch	Dinner	Bedtime
	Blood Pressure	/	/	/	/
	Blood Sugar				

Date	Test	Breakfast	Lunch	Dinner	Bedtime
	Blood Pressure	/	/	/	/
	Blood Sugar				

Date	Test	Breakfast	Lunch	Dinner	Bedtime
	Blood Pressure	/	/	/	/
	Blood Sugar				

Date	Test	Breakfast	Lunch	Dinner	Bedtime
	Blood Pressure	/	/	/	/
	Blood Sugar				

Date	Test	Breakfast	Lunch	Dinner	Bedtime
	Blood Pressure	/	/	/	/
	Blood Sugar				

Date	Test	Breakfast	Lunch	Dinner	Bedtime
	Blood Pressure	/	/	/	/
	Blood Sugar				

Date	Test	Breakfast	Lunch	Dinner	Bedtime
	Blood Pressure	/	/	/	/
	Blood Sugar				

Date	Test	Breakfast	Lunch	Dinner	Bedtime
	Blood Pressure	/	/	/	/
	Blood Sugar				

Date	Test	Breakfast	Lunch	Dinner	Bedtime
	Blood Pressure	/	/	/	/
	Blood Sugar				

Date	Test	Breakfast	Lunch	Dinner	Bedtime
	Blood Pressure	/	/	/	/
	Blood Sugar				

Date	Test	Breakfast	Lunch	Dinner	Bedtime
	Blood Pressure	/	/	/	/
	Blood Sugar				

Date	Test	Breakfast	Lunch	Dinner	Bedtime
	Blood Pressure	/	/	/	/
	Blood Sugar				

Date	Test	Breakfast	Lunch	Dinner	Bedtime
	Blood Pressure	/	/	/	/
	Blood Sugar				

Date	Test	Breakfast	Lunch	Dinner	Bedtime
	Blood Pressure	/	/	/	/
	Blood Sugar				

Date	Test	Breakfast	Lunch	Dinner	Bedtime
	Blood Pressure	/	/	/	/
	Blood Sugar				

Date	Test	Breakfast	Lunch	Dinner	Bedtime
	Blood Pressure	/	/	/	/
	Blood Sugar				

Date	Test	Breakfast	Lunch	Dinner	Bedtime
	Blood Pressure	/	/	/	/
	Blood Sugar				

Date	Test	Breakfast	Lunch	Dinner	Bedtime
	Blood Pressure	/	/	/	/
	Blood Sugar				

Date	Test	Breakfast	Lunch	Dinner	Bedtime
	Blood Pressure	/	/	/	/
	Blood Sugar				

Date	Test	Breakfast	Lunch	Dinner	Bedtime
	Blood Pressure	/	/	/	/
	Blood Sugar				

Date	Test	Breakfast	Lunch	Dinner	Bedtime
	Blood Pressure	/	/	/	/
	Blood Sugar				

Date	Test	Breakfast	Lunch	Dinner	Bedtime
	Blood Pressure	/	/	/	/
	Blood Sugar				

Date	Test	Breakfast	Lunch	Dinner	Bedtime
	Blood Pressure	/	/	/	/
	Blood Sugar				

Date	Test	Breakfast	Lunch	Dinner	Bedtime
	Blood Pressure	/	/	/	/
	Blood Sugar				

Date	Test	Breakfast	Lunch	Dinner	Bedtime
	Blood Pressure	/	/	/	/
	Blood Sugar				

Date	Test	Breakfast	Lunch	Dinner	Bedtime
	Blood Pressure	/	/	/	/
	Blood Sugar				

Date	Test	Breakfast	Lunch	Dinner	Bedtime
	Blood Pressure	/	/	/	/
	Blood Sugar				

Date	Test	Breakfast	Lunch	Dinner	Bedtime
	Blood Pressure	/	/	/	/
	Blood Sugar				

Date	Test	Breakfast	Lunch	Dinner	Bedtime
	Blood Pressure	/	/	/	/
	Blood Sugar				

Date	Test	Breakfast	Lunch	Dinner	Bedtime
	Blood Pressure	/	/	/	/
	Blood Sugar				

Date	Test	Breakfast	Lunch	Dinner	Bedtime
	Blood Pressure	/	/	/	/
	Blood Sugar				

Date	Test	Breakfast	Lunch	Dinner	Bedtime
	Blood Pressure	/	/	/	/
	Blood Sugar				

Date	Test	Breakfast	Lunch	Dinner	Bedtime
	Blood Pressure	/	/	/	/
	Blood Sugar				

Date	Test	Breakfast	Lunch	Dinner	Bedtime
	Blood Pressure	/	/	/	/
	Blood Sugar				

Date	Test	Breakfast	Lunch	Dinner	Bedtime
	Blood Pressure	/	/	/	/
	Blood Sugar				

Date	Test	Breakfast	Lunch	Dinner	Bedtime
	Blood Pressure	/	/	/	/
	Blood Sugar				

Date	Test	Breakfast	Lunch	Dinner	Bedtime
	Blood Pressure	/	/	/	/
	Blood Sugar				

Date	Test	Breakfast	Lunch	Dinner	Bedtime
	Blood Pressure	/	/	/	/
	Blood Sugar				

Date	Test	Breakfast	Lunch	Dinner	Bedtime
	Blood Pressure	/	/	/	/
	Blood Sugar				

Date	Test	Breakfast	Lunch	Dinner	Bedtime
	Blood Pressure	/	/	/	/
	Blood Sugar				

Date	Test	Breakfast	Lunch	Dinner	Bedtime
	Blood Pressure	/	/	/	/
	Blood Sugar				

Date	Test	Breakfast	Lunch	Dinner	Bedtime
	Blood Pressure	/	/	/	/
	Blood Sugar				

Date	Test	Breakfast	Lunch	Dinner	Bedtime
	Blood Pressure	/	/	/	/
	Blood Sugar				

Date	Test	Breakfast	Lunch	Dinner	Bedtime
	Blood Pressure	/	/	/	/
	Blood Sugar				

Date	Test	Breakfast	Lunch	Dinner	Bedtime
	Blood Pressure	/	/	/	/
	Blood Sugar				

Date	Test	Breakfast	Lunch	Dinner	Bedtime
	Blood Pressure	/	/	/	/
	Blood Sugar				

Date	Test	Breakfast	Lunch	Dinner	Bedtime
	Blood Pressure	/	/	/	/
	Blood Sugar				

Date	Test	Breakfast	Lunch	Dinner	Bedtime
	Blood Pressure	/	/	/	/
	Blood Sugar				

Date	Test	Breakfast	Lunch	Dinner	Bedtime
	Blood Pressure	/	/	/	/
	Blood Sugar				

Date	Test	Breakfast	Lunch	Dinner	Bedtime
	Blood Pressure	/	/	/	/
	Blood Sugar				

Date	Test	Breakfast	Lunch	Dinner	Bedtime
	Blood Pressure	/	/	/	/
	Blood Sugar				

Date	Test	Breakfast	Lunch	Dinner	Bedtime
	Blood Pressure	/	/	/	/
	Blood Sugar				

Date	Test	Breakfast	Lunch	Dinner	Bedtime
	Blood Pressure	/	/	/	/
	Blood Sugar				

Date	Test	Breakfast	Lunch	Dinner	Bedtime
	Blood Pressure	/	/	/	/
	Blood Sugar				

Date	Test	Breakfast	Lunch	Dinner	Bedtime
	Blood Pressure	/	/	/	/
	Blood Sugar				

Date	Test	Breakfast	Lunch	Dinner	Bedtime
	Blood Pressure	/	/	/	/
	Blood Sugar				

Date	Test	Breakfast	Lunch	Dinner	Bedtime
	Blood Pressure	/	/	/	/
	Blood Sugar				

Date	Test	Breakfast	Lunch	Dinner	Bedtime
	Blood Pressure	/	/	/	/
	Blood Sugar				

Date	Test	Breakfast	Lunch	Dinner	Bedtime
	Blood Pressure	/	/	/	/
	Blood Sugar				

Date	Test	Breakfast	Lunch	Dinner	Bedtime
	Blood Pressure	/	/	/	/
	Blood Sugar				

Date	Test	Breakfast	Lunch	Dinner	Bedtime
	Blood Pressure	/	/	/	/
	Blood Sugar				

Date	Test	Breakfast	Lunch	Dinner	Bedtime
	Blood Pressure	/	/	/	/
	Blood Sugar				

Date	Test	Breakfast	Lunch	Dinner	Bedtime
	Blood Pressure	/	/	/	/
	Blood Sugar				

Date	Test	Breakfast	Lunch	Dinner	Bedtime
	Blood Pressure	/	/	/	/
	Blood Sugar				

NOTE

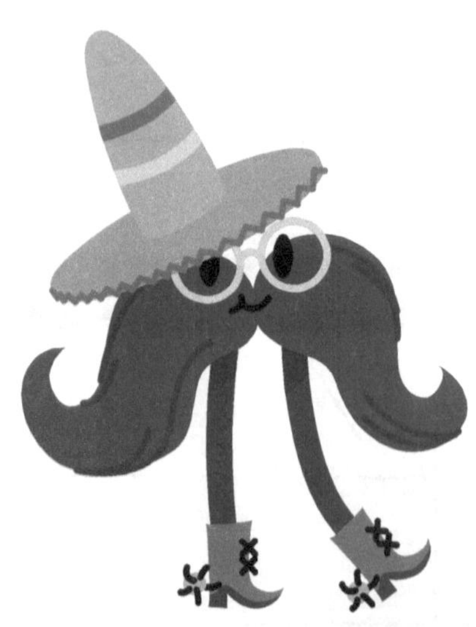

NOTE

NOTE

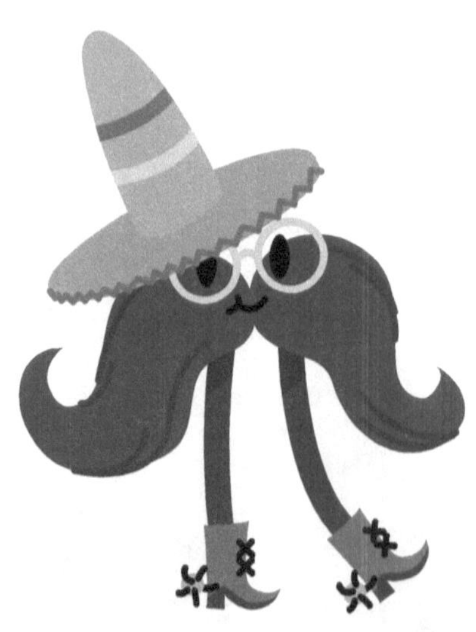

www.ingramcontent.com/pod-product-compliance
Lightning Source LLC
Chambersburg PA
CBHW031257250726
48655CB00005B/2255